Healthy Foods of the World

By Matthew Denny

Covers by Matde38
{MD}

ISBN-13: 978-1500821692

ISBN-10: 1500821691

Table of contents

A
Acai berry   2
Allspice   2
Almond   3
Amaranth   3
Apple   4
Apple cider vinegar   5
Artichoke   5
Apricot   6
Asafetida   6
Asian pear   7
Asparagus   7
Avocado   8

B
Bamboo   9
Banana   9
Barley   10
Basil   10
Bay leaf   11
Beans   11
Beet   12
Bell Pepper   12
Blackberry   13
Blackcurrant   13
Black Eyed Pea   14
Black Pepper   14
Blueberry   15
Bok Choy   15

Boniato root   16
Breadfruit   16
Broccoli   17
Brussels sprouts   17
Buckwheat   18
Bulgur   19

C

Cabbage   20
Cantaloupe   21
Caper   21
Cardamom   22
Caraway   22
Carrots   23
Cashew   23
Cauliflower   24
Celery   24
Chayote   25
Cherry   25
Chia   26
Chickpea   26
Chiles (hot peppers)   27
Chives   27
Chocolate (cocoa)   28
Cinnamon   29
Clove   29
Coconut   30
Coffee   30
Conkerberry   31
Coriander, Cilantro   31
Corn   32
Cranberry   32
Cucumber   33
Cumin   33
Currant   33

Curry Leaf   34

D
Dandelion   35
Date   35
Dill   36
Durian   36

E
Egg (chicken)   37
Eggplant   37
Endive   38
Epazote   38

F
Farro   40
Fennel   40
Fenugreek seeds   41
Fig   41
Flaxseed   42
Freekeh   42

G
Galangal   43
Garlic   43
Ginger   44
Gooseberry   44
Goumi   45
Grape   45
Grapefruit   46
Green beans   46
Guava   47

H

Hearts of palm   48
Horseradish   48
Honey   49
Huckleberry   49

I
Indian Gooseberry   50

J
Jackfruit   51
Jambul   51
Jicama   52
Jujube fruit   53
Jute leaves   53

K
Kale   54
Kiwifruit   54
Kohlrabi   55
Krachai   55
Kumquat   56

L
Lanzones   57
Leek   57
Lemon   57
Lemongrass   58
Lentils   58
Lettuce   59
Lime   59
Longan   60
Lychee (Litchi)   60

M

Macadamia Nut   61
Mace   61
Malanga   62
Mango   62
Mangosteen   63
Maygrass   63
Milk   64
Millet   64
Mint   65
Mulberry   65
Mushrooms   66
Mustard Seed   66

N
Nance   67
Nectarines   67
Nungu   67

O
Oats   69
Okra   70
Olive   70
Onion   70
Orange   71

P
Papaya   72
Parsley   72
Parsnip   73
Pawpaw   73
Peach   74
Peanut   74
Pear   75
Peas   75
Pecan   76

Persimmon   76
Pimento   77
Pineapple   77
Pine nuts   78
Pistachio   78
Pitaya fruit   79
Plantains   79
Plum   80
Pomegranate   80
Pomelo, Pummelo   81
Potato   81
Pumpkin   82
Purslane   83

Q
Quinoa   84

R
Radish   85
Rambutan   85
Rapini, broccoli rabe   86
Raspberry   86
Rhubarb   87
Rice   87
Rutabaga   88
Rye   88

S
Saffron   89
Sage   89
Sapodilla   90
Seaweed   90
Sesame   91
Sorghum   91
Soybean   92

Spelt	92
Spinach	93
Summer Squash	93
Star Anise	94
Star fruit	94
Strawberry	95
Sunflower seed	95
Sweet Potato	96
Swiss Chard	97

T

Tapioca	98
Taro	98
Tamarind	99
Tarragon	99
Tea	100
Teff	100
Tomatillo	101
Tomato	101
Triticale	102
Turmeric	103
Turnip	103

V

Vanilla	104

W

Walnut	105
Wasabi	106
Wasabi Plant	106
Water Chestnut	107
Watercress	107
Watermelon	107
Wheat	108
Wild Rice	109

Winter Squash   109

X
Ximenia   111

Y
Yam   112
Yautia   112
Yogurt   113
Yucca   113
Yuzu fruit   114

Anti-oxidants   115
Nutrients   117
Phytonutrients   128
Polyphenols   129

Preface

I have compiled a list of the foods that are good for the body and mind from around the world. The information for the foods in this book is a compilation of different areas of the world and different peoples. Because of this, the uses for the foods in this book may have wildly different uses that may even contradict. I have avoided adding herbs not commonly used for cooking or eating. There are many herbs and "foods" used solely for their medicinal purposes. Such foods and herbs are outside the scope of this book.

This book is not intended to treat, cure or prevent any disease. Instead this book is a listing of foods believed around the world to have healthy and healing properties. Some of these beliefs are from ancient cultures some from modern research; I do not make any distinction in this book.

Through my research for this book I have found that eating a balanced and varied diet of fruits and vegetables could provide all necessary vitamins and minerals. It is surprising how many fruits and vegetables can reduce the risk of cancer and lower cholesterol and blood pressure.

This book is not an all inclusive listing of the world's foods. There is ongoing research that may bring new light to some of the foods in this book and thus contradict with it. I have attempted to make this book as correct as possible with the current knowledge.

M. Denny

A

Acai Berry:

Acai berries are ranked the highest when it comes to antioxidants. They are high in protein and monounsaturated fats, yet are believed to help in weight loss. Acai berries are high in photochemicals that may help maintain the circulatory system, ensure proper nerve function and fight cancer. Acai berries are also high in omega-6 and omega-9 fatty acids which help reduce cholesterol.

High in:
Vitamin A
Calcium
Fiber

Allspice:

Allspice, also known as Jamaican pepper or pimento is the dried berry of a tropical evergreen. It is believed to have anti-inflammatory and anti-flatulent properties. Allspice is also considered to be warming and soothing in nature. It is believed that allspice improves digestion and increases enzyme secretions in the stomach and intestines. One teaspoon of allspice has 4-6 calories.

High in:
Manganese
Vitamin C
Calcium
Iron
Magnesium
Potassium

Almond:

Almonds are high in protein but have no Cholesterol making them healthy for the heart. Some of the nutrients in Almonds have been found to reduce cancer risks. Rhizveritrol the anti-inflammatory agent found in red wine is also found in Almonds. People who are allergic to Peaches they may also be allergic to Almonds. One Almond has 5-10 calories.

High in:
Unsaturated fats
Vitamin E
Protein
Magnesium
Copper
Calcium

Amaranth:

Amaranth is known as the "miracle grain" of the Aztecs, but is actually the seed of an herb. Amaranth can be used as a gluten free grain that is high in protein. The seeds can be ground into flour for baking or simmered in water to be used as a hot cereal. High in nutrition, Amaranth may help prevent chronic degenerative disease and may help reduce cholesterol. The leaves of the plant can also be used is soups. Amaranth oil is believed to help with hypertension and coronary heart disease. Amaranth seeds are high in fiber and low in saturated fats. One cup of amaranth seeds has 716 calories and 322% of recommended daily intake of manganese.

High in:
Thiamin
Riboflavin

Vitamin B6
Folate
Pantothenic acid
Iron
Magnesium
Phosphorus
Copper
Zinc
Manganese
Selenium

Apple:

Apples are high in fiber which can reduce your cholesterol. Lower cholesterol may help reduce the risk of heart disease. The Pectin in apples may help to remove harmful toxin from the body. Apples may also protect against certain types of cancer. They may also help to regulate blood sugar and reduce the risk of kidney stones. Reported to be good for the brain, apples may reduce the risk of Alzheimer's and Parkinson's diseases. There are roughly 110-120 calories in an apple.

High in:
Vitamin C
Fiber
Potassium

Apple Cider Vinegar:

Cider vinegar may help in weight loss by slowing the digestion of starches. It is said that a splash of vinegar will let you eat less at the next meal. The acids in cider vinegar may help in digestion. It is believed that cider vinegar has antiseptic properties that help deter bacterial and yeast growth in the digestive track. Unfiltered cider vinegar is best as it retains the vitamins and minerals present in apples. One tablespoon of vinegar has around 3 calories.

High in:
Manganese

Artichoke:

Artichokes are high in potassium which is believed to help maintain a normal heart rhythm. Potassium is reputed to tone down sodium and reduce the risk of stroke. Artichokes are high in antioxidants and vitamin C, which helps the immune system. They are also high in fiber which helps with digestion, blood health and weight control. The magnesium in artichokes may support the central nervous systems. One medium artichoke has 60-80 calories.

High in:
Vitamin C
Vitamin K
Folate
Magnesium
Phosphorus
Potassium
Copper
Manganese

Apricot:

Apricots are high in fiber and antioxidants, but low in calories. High in vitamin A and carotenes, apricots are good for the eyes as well as the skin. They are also high in potassium which helps regulate blood pressure. It is believed that the zea-xanthin in apricots may reduce the risk of age-related macular disease of the eyes. One apricot has 15-17 calories.

High in:
Vitamin A
Potassium
Vitamin C

Asafetida:

Asafetida is a dried resin from several species of giant fennel. It is thought to have anti-inflammatory, anti-oxidant and anti-microbial properties. Asafetida has been used to treat respiratory and emotional disorders. It has also been used to treat opium addiction and lower blood pressure. Asafetida is toxic to infants and in large doses. One 2 gram serving has 3-5 calories.

High in:
Calcium
Phosphorous
Iron

Asian Pear:

Asian pear has vitamins, minerals and fiber. Most of the calories are in the form of sugars. One Asian pear has 50-60 calories.

High in:
Vitamin C
Vitamin K
Potassium

Asparagus:

Asparagus is high in vitamins and fiber. It is believed to have healthy benefits for the lower digestive tract. Asparagus does not store well and should be eaten soon after harvesting. Some people may experience a pungent odor from their urine after eating asparagus; this is caused by enzymes in the body and is harmless. One cup of asparagus has 30-40 calories.

High in:
Vitamin A
Vitamin C
Vitamin E
Vitamin K
Folate
Riboflavin
Manganese
Selenium

Avocado:

Avocadoes are high in unsaturated fats that are said to reduce blood cholesterol. Avocados have nearly twenty vitamins and minerals. They are also believed to be good for bones, skin and muscles because of their antioxidants. Avocados are also believed to help reduce the risk of eye disease. One fifth of a medium avocado has 45-55 calories.

High in:
Vitamin K
Folate

B

Bamboo:

Bamboo adds bulk and texture to food without adding a lot of fat and calories. Bamboo is high in fiber and potassium. One bamboo shoot has 15-20 calories.

High in:
Vitamin B6
Fiber
Potassium
Sodium
Zinc
Copper
Manganese

Banana:

Bananas are naturally fat and cholesterol free and high in fiber and potassium. Bananas are believed to have an antacid effect and may be able to reduce the effects of diarrhea. It is also believed that bananas can improve eyesight and build stronger bones. One medium banana has 100-120 calories.

High in:
Vitamin C
Vitamin B6
Potassium
Manganese

Barley:

Barley is high in fiber that may help in lowering cholesterol and protecting the digestive tract. The fiber in barley is said to feed beneficial bacteria in the intestines. This bacterium helps the liver and muscles of the digestive tract. It is also believed that barley can reduce the risk of type 2 diabetes and prevent heart failure. It is thought that barley can help prevent breast cancer and gallstones. One cup of barley has 190-210 calories.

High in:
Niacin
Iron
Fiber
Magnesium
Phosphorus
Zinc
Copper
Manganese
Selenium

Basil:

Basil is very high in vitamin K and has anti-inflammatory and anti-bacterial properties. Basil is also a good source of vitamin A and beta-carotene. It also has essential nutrients for cardiovascular health. It is believed that basil can protect the body at the cellular level. Two tablespoons of fresh chopped basil leaves has around one calorie.

High in:
Vitamin K
Vitamin A
Vitamin C
Manganese

Bay Leaf:

Bay leaf is believed to have anti-oxidant and anti-cancer properties. It also has astringent, diuretic and appetite stimulant properties. Bay leaves have also been used to soothe the stomach and relieve flatulence. One teaspoon of crumbled bay leaf has 1-3 calories.

High in:
Manganese
Vitamin A
Fiber
Iron

Beans:

Beans are low in fat and high in protein and potassium. They are high in soluble fiber which lowers blood cholesterol and may prevent degenerative diseases. The potassium and magnesium in beans may help to lower blood pressure and improve blood flow. Beans are high in nutrients that may help reduce the risk of cancer, heart disease and anemia. Bean may also aid in heart and bone health and sooth the nervous system. One cup of beans has 140-250 calories.

High in:
Potassium
Iron
Thiamine

Folate
Zinc
Copper
Manganese

Beet:

Beets are low in calories and fat and have no cholesterol. The root is high in phytochemicals that are believed to reduce toxins in the blood and reduce the risk of coronary disease. Raw beets are high in Folate; but over cooking may deplete this vitamin. The greens are very high in vitamin C whereas the root has only a small amount. Some people may have pink urine or excreatment after eating beets which is harmless. One beet has 30-40 calories.

High in:
Vitamin C
Folate
Potassium
Manganese

Bell Pepper:

Bell peppers are high in vitamin C and carotenoids which increase with the ripeness of the fruit. High temperature cooking can damage the nutrients in bell peppers. Bell peppers are also high nutrients than may have anti-oxidant and anti-inflammatory properties. It is believed that these nutrients may have anti-cancer abilities. One medium bell pepper has 20-30 calories.

High in:
Vitamin C
Vitamin K

Vitamin B6
Potassium
Manganese

Blackberry:

Blackberries are an aggregate fruit made up of many smaller berries, this adds to the fiber content. They are also high in anti-oxidants. Historically, blackberries have been used to treat infections of the mouth and eyes. One cup of blackberries has 55-65 calories.

High in:
Vitamin C
Vitamin K
Fiber
Copper
Manganese

Blackcurrant:

Blackcurrants are high in anti-oxidants and vitamins. They also have anti-inflammatory properties. It is believed that blackcurrants may prevent cancer and lessen the effects of arthritis. One cup of blackcurrants has 65-75 calories.

High in:
Vitamin C
Iron
Potassium
Manganese

Black Eyed Pea:

Black eyed peas are high in vitamins and protein as well as fiber. They are actually beans. Black eyed peas are believed to be able to reduce cholesterol and regulate blood sugar. One cup of black eyed peas has 180-210 calories.

High in:
Thiamin
Fiber
Folate
Pantothenic acid
Iron
Magnesium
Phosphorus
Copper
Manganese

Black Pepper:

Black pepper is said to stimulate the stomach to increase the production of acid; aiding in digestion. It is thought that black pepper can prevent the formation of intestinal gas. Black pepper is believed to have strong anti-oxidant and anti-bacterial properties. One teaspoon of black pepper has 4-6 calories.

High in:
Vitamin K
Iron
Manganese

Blueberry:

Blueberries have among the highest levels of anti-oxidants. Blueberries have multiple types of anti-oxidants. It is believed that blueberries have the ability to lower blood sugar levels and control blood glucose levels. One cup of blueberries has 80-90 calories.

High in:
Vitamin C
Vitamin K
Manganese
Fiber

Bok Choy (Chinese cabbage):

Bok Choy is high in vitamins, minerals and anti-oxidants, but is low in calories. It is believed that Bok Choy requires more calories to digest than are gained. Bok Choy may help create a resistance to infectious agents, such as cold and flu germs. One cup of Bok Choy has 15-30 calories.

High in:
Vitamin A
Vitamin C
Vitamin K
Vitamin B6
Folate
Calcium
Iron
Potassium
Manganese

Boniato root:

The Boniato is an ancient type of sweet potato. Boniato is rich in vitamin C and fiber and low in sodium. One small Boniato root has 90-110 calories.

High in:
Fiber
Vitamin C

Breadfruit:

Breadfruit is high in vitamins and minerals, but also high in calories. They have some anti-oxidant properties. Breadfruit is an excellent source of vitamin C and potassium. The seeds have some protein as well. One cup of breadfruit has 220-230 calories.

High in:
Vitamin C
Thiamin
Niacin
Fiber
Vitamin B6
Pantothenic acid
Magnesium
Potassium

Broccoli:

Broccoli is believed to have a strong effect on the body's detoxification system. The phytonutrients in broccoli may be able to help with activation, neutralization, and elimination of unwanted contaminants in the body. The vitamin A and Vitamin K in broccoli may help to rebuild vitamin D levels with the use of supplements. Eating broccoli may reduce the effects of allergies. Broccoli has anti-inflammatory properties as well as being able to reduce oxidative stress. This may reduce the risk of getting some cancers. Broccoli may also support the cardiovascular and digestive systems. It has been shown in studies that microwaving broccoli can destroy up to 90 percent of the nutrients therein. One cup of chopped broccoli has 25-35 calories.

High in:
Vitamin A
Vitamin C
Vitamin K
Folate
Manganese

Brussels sprouts:

Brussels sprouts are high in vitamins C and K. They are also low in calories. It is believed that Brussels sprouts can reduce the risk of getting cancer. One sprout has 6-9 calories.

High in:
Vitamin C
Vitamin K
Folate
Vitamin A
Potassium
Manganese

Buckwheat:

Buckwheat is a fruit seed that is related to rhubarb and is gluten free substitute for grains. A diet high in buckwheat may lower blood cholesterol and blood pressure. Buckwheat may also control blood sugar levels and improve insulin response. High fiber foods such as buckwheat may reduce the risk of gallstones. It is believed that buckwheat may have more cancer preventing abilities than fruits and vegetables. One cup of buckwheat has 570-590 calories and 111% of recommended daily intake of manganese.

High In:
Thiamin
Riboflavin
Niacin
Vitamin B6
Pantothenic acid
Iron
Magnesium
Phosphorus
Potassium
Zinc
Copper
Manganese
Selenium

Bulgur:

Bulgur is a grain from the Middle East and is low in fat and calories. It is high in protein and fiber. Bulgur has anti-inflammatory properties. It is believed that bulgur may reduce the risk of certain diseases such as; heart disease, osteoporosis, Alzheimer's and type 2 diabetes. Bulgur may also reduce the risk of gallstones. One cup of bulgur has 145-155 calories.

High in:
Manganese
Fiber
Magnesium
Protein

C

Cabbage:

The fiber in cabbage is believed to lower cholesterol and it is believed that this fiber is more effective after steaming. Different cabbages have different patterns in nutrients and a diet including red, green and Savoy would be beneficial. Savoy cabbage is believed to be especially good at preventing cancer. It is inadvisable to microwave cabbage because it may destroy the cancer preventing compounds. Cabbages also have anti-oxidant and anti-inflammatory properties. Historically the cabbage has been used to help with ulcers and other digestive tract problems. One medium head of cabbage has 200-230 calories.

High in:
Vitamin C
Vitamin K
Thiamin
Vitamin B6
Folate
Pantothenic acid
Calcium
Iron
Magnesium
Phosphorus
Potassium
Zinc
Manganese
Fiber

Cantaloupe:

Cantaloupes are high in vitamins A and C. They also have a high level of carotenoids. Cantaloupes have anti-oxidant and anti-inflammatory properties. It is believed that cantaloupes can reduce the risk of metabolic syndrome. One wedge of a medium melon has 20-30 calories.

High in:
Vitamin A
Vitamin C

Caper:

Capers are a flowering bud of a low growing shrub. Capers are high in powerful anti-oxidants and are believed to lower blood pressure. They may also be able to lower bad cholesterol levels. Historically capers have been used to relieve rheumatic pain and digestive problems. One tablespoon of capers has 1-3 calories.

High in:
Vitamin K
Riboflavin
Sodium
Copper
Iron

Cardamom:

Cardamom is a seed pod historically known for its' culinary and medicinal purposes. Cardamom is believed to have anti-oxidant properties as well as the ability to prevent disease and promote general health. One teaspoon of cardamom has 5-7 calories.

High in:
Vitamin C
Iron
Manganese

Caraway:

Caraway is the chief spice used in savory dishes in Europe. They are high in fiber and are believed to reduce intestinal transit time. Caraway seed are believed to reduce toxins and cholesterol in the blood. The essential oils in caraway seeds are believed to improve digestion. One teaspoon of caraway seeds has 6-8 calories.

High in:
Fiber
Vitamin C
Thiamin
Iron

Carrots:

Carrots help to reduce the risk of cardiovascular disease. They are high in antioxidants. Carrots are reputed to taste better if steamed. They are noted for being good for the eyes and to have anti-cancer properties. Overeating of carrots may turn the skin yellow or orange. The tops are edible and may be too tough to eat raw. Some people may have an allergic reaction to too much carrot greens. One medium carrot has 20-30 calories and 204% of daily recommended intake of vitamin A.

High in:
Vitamin A
Vitamin K
Fiber

Cashew:

Cashews are high in fatty acids, fiber, vitamins and minerals. Cashews are believed to be able to reduce the risk of many diseases, especially deficiency diseases. One ounce of cashews has 150-160 calories.

High in:
Protein
Vitamin K
Vitamin B6
Iron
Magnesium
Phosphorus
Zinc
Copper
Manganese

Cauliflower:

Cauliflower can provide support for level 1 and 2 detoxifications. It may also reduce the risk of getting cancer. Cauliflower is believed to have anti-oxidant and anti-inflammatory properties. It is also believed that cauliflower supports the cardiovascular and digestive systems. The nutrients in cauliflower can be damaged from over cooking. One cup of cauliflower has 20-30 calories.

High in:
Protein
Vitamin C
Vitamin K
Vitamin B6
Folate
Potassium
Manganese

Celery:

Celery has multiple types of anti-oxidants and has anti-inflammatory properties. Celery is believed to be good for the digestive tract and the cardiovascular system. Being low in calories and high in fiber, it may be that celery requires more calories to digest than are obtained from eating. One medium stalk of celery has 6-7 calories.

High in:
Vitamin A
Vitamin K
Fiber
Calcium
Potassium
Sodium

Manganese

Chayote:

Chayote also known as mirliton is a pear shaped member of the gourd family. Chayote is believed to be good for lowering cholesterol and body weight. They are also a good source of anti-oxidants. One chayote has 35-45 calories.

High in:
Vitamin C
Vitamin K
Folate
Zinc
Copper
Manganese
Fiber

Cherry:

Tart cherries are believed to help with insomnia. They May also help reduce post workout pain. Tart cherries may also increase the metabolism and reduce the amount of fat stored by the body. Sweet cherries may be able to regulate blood pressure and help fight cancer. Cherries both tart and sweet may reduce the symptoms of gout by reducing the amount of uric acid in the body. One cup of cherries has 80-90 calories.

High in:
Vitamin C
Potassium
Fiber

Chia:

Chia is edible seed that come from a desert plant. Chia seeds are high in omega-3 fatty acids as well as other important nutrients. They were grown in ancient Mexico by the Mayans and Aztecs. It is believed that Chia seeds can help with weight loss by expanding in the stomach. Chia seeds are the same that come with Chia Pets and can be harvested from them. One tablespoon of Chia seeds 60-70 calories.

High in:
Fiber
Protein
Calcium
Phosphorus
Manganese

Chickpea:

Chickpeas, otherwise known as garbanzo beans, are high in a fiber believed to reduce cholesterol and support the colon. One cup of chickpeas has 50% of your daily value of fiber; to thirds of which is insoluble. They are also high in valuable anti-oxidants. Chickpeas may be able to regulate blood sugar and help with weight loss. One cup of chickpeas has 250-270 calories.

High in:
Protein
Fiber
Thiamin
Vitamin B6
Folate
Iron
Magnesium
Phosphorus

Copper
Manganese

Chilies (hot peppers):

Chiles can be used for weight loss. The capsaicin in chilies can increase the metabolism as much as 25%. The "heat" can also deter over eating, if many chilies are used. They are actually a fruit. Capsaicin is reported to reduce the risk of cancer. Some people believe capsaicin can even cure cancer. Capsaicin is also used in topical ointments to relieve pain. It is believed that capsaicin can reduce the cholesterol in the blood and in blood vessels. The calories in chilies depend upon size and the heat depends upon the levels of capsaicin.

High in:
Vitamin A
Vitamin C
Capsaicin

Chives:

Chives are high in vitamins and minerals but very low in calories. They are a member of the Lilly family. They are very high in vitamin K which is believed to help treat Alzheimer's disease. One tablespoon of chives has 0-1 calories.

High in:
Vitamin A
Vitamin C
Vitamin K

Chocolate (Cocoa):

Cocoa is believed to lower blood pressure and reduce the bloods ability to clot. Cocoa has anti-oxidants, caffeine and theobromine. Theobromine is a diuretic that is toxic to dogs, cats and parrots. It may help to relive the symptoms of depression and PMS. Cocoa also has essential vitamins and minerals. It is believed that cocoa increases blood flow through the brain, this may help treat Alzheimer's and Parkinson's diseases. One cup of cocoa powder has 190-200 calories.

Milk adds fat and calories to cocoa. Dark chocolate is the better source for cocoa than milk chocolate.

High in:
Riboflavin
Phosphorus
Manganese
Iron
Potassium
Zinc
Copper

Cinnamon:

Cinnamon may help to metabolize sugar in the food and may control cravings for sweets. It has been reported that cinnamon has anti-inflammatory and anti-fungal properties. Cinnamon has been used as a treatment for digestive tract problems as well as food preservation. It has even been reported that sniffing cinnamon can improve brain function. Cinnamon has been shown to increase insulin sensitivity and blood glucose control; which would help with weight control. In high doses cinnamon can cause skin irritation or bleeding problems in people who take medications that thin the blood. One teaspoon of cinnamon has 4-7 calories.

High in:
Manganese
Calcium
Iron

Clove:

Cloves are a flower bud from an evergreen tree. They are believed to be able to relive indigestion and constipation. Clove is also thought to have anti-oxidant, anti-septic, anti-inflammatory and anti-flatulent properties. One tablespoon of ground clove has 20-25 calories.

High in:
Vitamin C
Vitamin K
Calcium
Manganese
Iron

Coconut:

Coconuts are known to have lauric acid which is believed to have antifungal, antibacterial and antiviral properties. Fresh coconut juice is very high in electrolytes and can prevent dehydration during cases of diarrhea or strenuous exercise. Coconut oil contains medium chain triglycerides (MTC), which is an easily digested fatty acid that is said to increase the body's metabolism. Coconuts are believed to lower cholesterol and promote healthy thyroid function. One cup of coconut has 280-290 calories and 119% daily recommended intake of saturated fat.

High in:
Vitamin C
Thiamin
Folate
Pantothenic acid
Iron
Magnesium
Phosphorus
Potassium
Zinc
Copper
Manganese
Selenium

Coffee:

Coffee is a low calorie beverage as long as it is not "lightened" with creams and sugars. Coffee is believed to be able to reduce the risk of type 2 diabetes and Alzheimer's. Coffee is also high in anti-oxidants. It is thought that more than 3 cups of coffee a day may increase blood pressure. One cup of plain coffee has 1-2 calories.

High in:
Caffeine

Conkerberry:

Conkerberry is a plum like berry native to Australia. They are believed to have anti-oxidant and anti-cancer properties.

High in:
Vitamin C
Vitamin K

Coriander, Cilantro:

Cilantro contains no cholesterol but is rich in anti-oxidants, vitamins and some minerals. Both the plant (cilantro) and the seeds (coriander) have essential oils believed to promote good health. Cilantro is believed to help lower cholesterol levels. In traditional medicine it is believed that coriander seeds can be used as an analgesic, aphrodisiac, anti-spasmodic, deodorant, anti- fungal, weight loss, and a digestive aid. It is also believed that the leaves and stems are anti-septic and prevents gas. One quarter cup of cilantro leaves has 1-2 calories.

High in:
Vitamin A
Vitamin K

Corn:

Anti-oxidants can be found in all corn colors, but yellow corn has the highest amount. Corn is used as a staple food around the world. It is high in vitamins and minerals as well as fiber, protein and carbohydrates. It is believed that drying corn does not harm its anti-oxidant properties. One cup of corn has 600-620 calories.

High in:
Fiber
Vitamin A
Thiamin
Riboflavin
Niacin
Vitamin B6
Iron
Magnesium
Phosphorus
Zinc
Copper
Selenium
Protein

Cranberry:

Cranberries are believed to have the ability to prevent unary tract infections. They are also believed to have anti-oxidant, anti-inflammatory and anti-cancer properties. It is believed that eating whole fresh cranberries is more healthful than extracts or dried. One cup of cranberries has 45-55 calories.

High in:
Vitamin C
Fiber

Manganese

Cucumber:

Cucumbers are believed to reduce the risk of cardiovascular diseases and some cancers. They may have anti-oxidant and anti-inflammatory properties. One half cup of cucumber slices has 7-8 calories.

High in:
Vitamin K

Cumin:

Traditionally cumin seeds have been used to benefit the digestive and immune systems. Cumin seeds may also prevent certain cancers. They may also be able to help detoxify the body and help with general body maintenance. One teaspoon of cumin seeds has 10-20 calories.

High in:
Iron
Manganese
Calcium
Magnesium

Currant:

Currants are high in vitamin C and anti-oxidants. They also have a rare version of omega 6. One cup of currants has 60-70 calories.

High in:
Vitamin C
Vitamin K
Fiber
Potassium
Manganese

Curry Leaf:

Curry leaves are high in vitamins and minerals but have very few calories. Curry leaf powder is believed to reduce stress on pancreatic cells. Curry leaves are believed to have antioxidants and anti-inflammatory properties. They are also believed to purify the blood and fight cancer. Curry leaves have also been used in weight loss, improve eyesight, ease insomnia, and relieve heartburn and indigestion. It has been reported that curry leaves can be used to manage type 2 diabetes. Curry leaf has no discernable calories.

High in:
Vitamin A
Phosphorus
Iron
Fiber

D

Dandelion:

Dandelions are often thought of as a weed, they are however a herb. All parts of the plant can be used. The leaves are high in fiber and are believed to help reduce weight and control cholesterol levels in the blood. The root is used for various therapeutic uses. The leaves are rich in vitamin A and very rich in vitamin K. One cup of chopped dandelion greens has 20-30 calories and over 500% of daily recommended intake of vitamin K.

High In:
Vitamin K
Vitamin A
Vitamin C
Calcium
Iron
Manganese

Date:

Dates are high in fiber and simple sugars. They have anti-inflammatory and anti-infective properties. Dates are thought to be good for the eyes and the blood. They also may reduce the risk of some cancers. One date has 60-70 calories.

High in:
Fiber
Potassium
Copper
Manganese

Dill:

Dill contains no cholesterol and few calories, but has anti-oxidant properties. Dill has large amounts of vitamins and minerals, like other foods, but not the calories. Dill is believed to lower blood sugar levels. One cup of dill sprigs has 2-6 calories.

High in:
Vitamin A
Vitamin C
Manganese

Durian:

Durian has a unique penetrating odor and is outlawed on many public transportation systems. The seeds are also edible after being boiled. The flesh is made of simple sugars and is easily digestible. Durian is also a good source of vitamins, minerals and fiber. One cup of chopped durian has 340-370 calories.

High in:
Vitamin C
Thiamin
Riboflavin
Niacin
Vitamin B6
Folate
Magnesium
Potassium
Copper
Manganese

E

Egg (chicken):

Eggs have vitamins, minerals and high quality protein. Eggs are believed to be good for the brain and eyes. They are also recommended for pregnant women. One large egg has 77 calories.

High in:
Cholesterol
Protein
Riboflavin
Selenium
Vitamin D

Eggplant:

The anti-oxidants in eggplants may have a protective effect for brain cells. Eggplants have one of the most potent free radical scavengers found in plants. This compound is believed to have anti-cancer, anti-microbial, anti-viral and cholesterol lowering properties. Eggplants are believed to be able to lower blood cholesterol and arterial cholesterol. One cup of eggplant cubes has 30-40 calories.

High in:
Vitamin K
Vitamin B6
Sodium
Manganese
Fiber

Endive:

Endive is high in nutrients and low in calories. High in fiber, endive is believed to reduce blood glucose and cholesterol. Endive is also a good source of vitamin A and vitamin B complexes as well as many minerals. One head of endive has 70-80 calories and 1481% of daily recommended intake of vitamin K.

High in:
Vitamin A
Vitamin C
Vitamin K
Folate
Pantothenic acid
Calcium
Iron
Magnesium
Potassium
Zinc
Copper
Manganese
Fiber

Epazote:

Epazote is used to add a musky flavor to Mexican and other Latin American cooking. It has been more often thought of as a medicinal herb rather than a culinary one. Epazote is very low in calories and has no fat or cholesterol. The herb is used for stomach and intestinal aliments. It may also cure indigestion, cramps and ulcers. Epazote may have anti-diabetic and anti-cancer properties. Pregnant and nursing women should avoid this herb. One sprig of epazote has around one calorie.

High in:
Manganese
Folate
Magnesium
Calcium
Fiber

F

Farro:

Farro is one of the world's oldest grains. It is low in fat and has no cholesterol. Farro does have protein and a large amount of selenium. It is thought to have anti-cancer properties. Farro is also believed to have muscle relaxing abilities. One hundred grams of farro has 190-210 calories.

High in:
Selenium
Protein
Fiber
Phosphorus

Fennel:

Fennel is believed to have strong anti-oxidant and anti-cancer properties. Fennel also contains a vitamin C that is anti-microbial and supports the immune system. The fiber in fennel may be able to reduce blood cholesterol levels and support colon health. One cup of fennel slices has 25-35 calories.

High in:
Vitamin C
Potassium
Fiber

Fenugreek seeds:

Traditionally fenugreek has been used to cure digestion problems and improve lactation in women. Fenugreek is believed to lower blood cholesterol and help remove toxins from the body. It is thought that fenugreek may reduce blood sugar levels and help with insulin secretion. One tablespoon of fenugreek seeds has 30-40 calories.

High in:
Iron
Fiber

Fig:

Figs are high in vitamins and minerals and low in calories. They also provide fiber and anti-oxidants. It is believed that figs can lower blood sugar levels and control blood glucose levels. Figs are reported to reduce the risk of cancers, diabetes and degenerative diseases. One dried fig has 15-25 calories.

High in:
Vitamin K
Calcium
Iron
Magnesium
Phosphorus
Potassium
Copper
Manganese
Fiber

Flaxseed:

Also known as linseed, flaxseed is a good source for minerals, anti-oxidants and omega 3. Flaxseed is high in energy and dietary fiber. It is one of the top vegetable sources of omega 3 fatty acids. It is believed that eating flaxseed on a regular basis may reduce cholesterol and help prevent coronary artery disease. Flaxseeds have multiple nutrients that are believed to have anti-cancer and anti-inflammatory properties. One tablespoon of whole flaxseed has 50-60 calories.

High in:
Thiamin
Magnesium
Manganese
Fiber
Protein

Freekeh:

Freekeh is made from green wheat that has been dried and roasted. Freekeh is high in protein and fiber as well as vitamins and minerals. It is believed to have anti-oxidant properties and may prevent age related macular degeneration disease. It may help in weight loss by being filling, thus reducing the amount of food consumed. Freekeh is also thought to improve bowel health. One half cup of cooked Freekeh has 85-100 calories.

High in:
Protein
Fiber
Calcium
Iron
Potassium

G

Galangal:

Galangal is a rhizome similar to ginger and turmeric. It looks and tastes like ginger. Galangal is believed to treat nausea, flatulence, and dyspepsia. It also has anti-inflammatory, anti-oxidant and anticancer properties. Galangal may inhibit fatty-acid synthase which may reduce triglycerides and cholesterol. Two thirds of a cup of galangal has 55-65 calories.

High in:
Vitamin A
Vitamin C
Iron
Fiber
Sodium

Garlic:

Garlic is rich in a variety of sulfur containing compounds, which may help with iron uptake and controlling blood pressure. Garlic is believed to be able to lower blood sugar and total cholesterol. Garlic has antioxidant and anti-inflammatory properties. This allows garlic to protect blood cells and blood vessels. Garlic may be able to prevent clots from forming in the blood vessels. Garlic is also believed to have antibacterial and antiviral properties. It is possible that garlic protects against certain types of cancer if eaten daily or even weekly. One clove of garlic has 4-5 calories.

High in:
Vitamin B6
Vitamin C

Manganese

Ginger:

Historically ginger has been used to relieve the symptoms of gastrointestinal distress. It is also believed to be able to inhibit the formation of inflammatory compounds and have direct anti-inflammatory properties. Ginger has been used to reduce nausea and vomiting, especially during pregnancy. Ginger is believed to have anti-cancer properties. One teaspoon of ginger has 1-3 calories.

High in:
Potassium
Vitamin C
Magnesium
Copper
Manganese

Gooseberry:

Gooseberries are high in vitamin A and have been used to treat eye problems. They also have a significant amount of anti-oxidants. Gooseberries are thought to be good for the blood sugar levels and blood pressure. Gooseberries can be cooked without damaging the vitamin C content. One cup of gooseberries has 60-70 calories.

High in:
Vitamin A
Vitamin C
Fiber
Manganese

Goumi:

Goumi seed are edible and contain fiber. They are believed to be able to reduce cholesterol. Historically goumi has been used to treat diarrhea. It is believed that pregnant women should not eat goumi berries. They have the highest amount of Lycopene than any other fruit. One cup of goumi has 90-110 calories.

High in:
Vitamin A
Vitamin C
Vitamin E

Grape:

Grapes are called "the queen of fruits" in some cultures. They come in three main varieties; white/green, red/purple, and blue/black. Grapes are rich in resveratrol which is one of the most powerful antioxidants. Resveratrol may help reduce the risk of colon and prostate cancers, coronary heart disease, Alzheimer's and degenerative nerve disease. Grapes also are believed to have antiviral and antifungal properties. The antioxidants in grapes are concentrated in the skins and edible seeds. Grapes are a good source of many vitamins and minerals and are low in calories. One cup of grapes has 100-110 calories.

Red Grapes are abundant in anthocyanins; an antioxidant believed to have anti-allergic, anti-inflammatory, anti-microbial and anti-cancer properties. White grapes have a similar compound called catechins.

High in:
Vitamin C

Vitamin K
Potassium
Copper
Iron
Manganese

Grapefruit:

Grapefruit is high in Vitamin A, beta-carotene and Lycopene. It is believed that the pectin in grapefruit may reduce the risk of some cancers. It may also reduce blood cholesterol and overall cholesterol. Grapefruits may be good for the skin, mucus membranes, the eyes and lungs. Red grapefruits may also prevent cancers of the skin and prostate. One half grapefruit has 45-55 calories.

High in:
Vitamin A
Vitamin C
Fiber
Potassium

Green beans:

Green beans are fat free and high in fiber. It is believed that green beans can reduce the risk of some cancers. Green beans may also support the skin, eyes and digestive system. One cup of green beans has 30-40 calories.

High in:
Fiber
Vitamin A
Vitamin C
Vitamin K
Folate
Manganese

Guava:

Guava is low in calories and fats but high in vitamins and minerals. They are believed to have anti-cancer, anti-aging, anti-oxidant, and immune boosting properties. Guava is believed to be able to help remove toxins from the body. They also contain more potassium than bananas by weight. One cup of raw guava has 100-120 calories and 628% of daily recommended intake of vitamin C.

High in:
Vitamin A
Vitamin C
Folate
Potassium
Copper
Manganese
Fiber

H

Hearts of Palm:

Hearts of palm are smooth and firm, and described as tasting like artichoke. They are low in calories and fat free. Hearts of palm are high in vitamins, minerals and fiber. One cup of hearts of palm has 35-45 calories and 102% of daily recommended intake of manganese.

High in:
Fiber
Protein
Vitamin C
Folate
Iron
Magnesium
Sodium
Zinc
Copper
Manganese

Honey:

Honey is 80% sugar but has a low GI, so will not spick blood sugar levels. It is believed that honey can help metabolize cholesterol and fats on the organs of the body. Honey is a better sweetener than table sugar for diabetics and non-diabetics alike. Honey is not recommended for children under one year of age. It is believed that eating local honey may reduce summer allergies. Honey is also thought to have anti-oxidant properties. One cup of honey has 1020-1040 calories.

High in:

Iron
Manganese

Horseradish:

Historically horseradish has been used to relieve dental ailments and treat scurvy. Horseradish may be help in treating sinus infections by thinning the mucus in the nasal cavities. Horseradish can also help relieving the symptoms of lung congestion and influenza. Horseradish also has anti-cancer and anti-biotic properties. One tablespoon of prepared horseradish has 5-10 calories.

High in:
Vitamin C
Fiber
Folate
Sodium

Huckleberry:

Huckleberries are higher in anti-oxidants than almost any other fruit or vegetable. They are thought to help the pancreas digest sugars and starches. The dried leaves of huckleberries can be made into a tea to treat digestive issues. Huckleberries may help in eye function and promote insulin production in diabetics. Huckleberries have been used as a laxative and to treat diarrhea. One tablespoon of huckleberries has 5-15 calories.

High in:
Vitamin C
Vitamin A
Niacin
Calcium
Sodium

I

Indian Gooseberry:

Historically Indian gooseberries have been used to treat conjunctivitis and to protect against diseases. They are believed to be good for the eyes and the liver. Indian gooseberries have also been used as a relaxant and sedative. One cup of Indian gooseberries has 50 -70 calories.

High in:
Vitamin C
Calcium
Fiber

J

Jackfruit:

Jackfruit has no cholesterol or saturated fats and is one of the largest tree-borne fruits. Jackfruit has simple sugars that replenish energy quickly. Jackfruit is rich in fiber and anti-oxidants. The seed are also rich in proteins and nutrients. One cup of jackfruit slices has 150-160 calories.

High in:
Vitamin C
Riboflavin
Potassium
Copper
Manganese
Fiber

Jambul:

Jambul is also known as the monsoon fruit although it is now grown around the world. It is believed to treat piles, diabetes, diarrhea, dysentery, sterility and liver problems. The seeds of the jambul are believed to increase the insulin production if the pancreas. The seeds can be dried and powdered and used to treat diarrhea and dysentery as well as other diseases. The jambul should not be eaten is excess as it can cause throat and chest problems. One cup of jambul has 75-85 calories.

High in:
Vitamin A
Vitamin B6
Vitamin C
Niacin

Iron

Jicama:

Jicama, also known as the yam bean is a taproot vegetable of the bean family with an inedible skin. Jicama is low in calories but high in anti-oxidants, fiber and some vitamins and minerals. They have a sweet inert carbohydrate that does not metabolize in the human body, which makes it an ideal sweet snack for diabetics and dieters. The skin has an organic poison and should be discarded. One medium jicama has 240-260 calories and 222% of daily recommended intake of vitamin C and 129% of fiber.

High in:
Vitamin C
Fiber
Vitamin E
Riboflavin
Folate
Iron
Magnesium
Phosphorus
Potassium
Copper
Manganese

Jujube fruit:

Jujube fruit also known as the Chinese date has more vitamin C than any other citrus fruits. They also have 18 out of the 24 important amino acids. Jujube fruit is believed to help healing and improves overall immune system function. They are also believed to be able to lower blood pressure and stress. Jujube fruit are rich in anti-oxidants and anti-cancer nutrients. They have been used in traditional medicine to improve immune system, relieve sore throats, purify the blood, and to aid digestion. One ounce of raw jujube fruit has 20-25 calories.

High in:
Vitamin C
Potassium

Jute leaves:

Jute leaves also known as saluyot is used to thicken soups and stews. One cup of jute leaves has 5-15 calories.

High in:
Vitamin A
Vitamin C

K

Kale:

Kale is low in calories but rich in vitamins and minerals. Kale is believed to have anti-oxidant, anti-cancer and anti-inflammatory properties. Kale is thought to lower cholesterol levels in the body. Kale is also believed to help the body detoxify itself, thus protecting it from toxic exposure in the environment and from food. Steaming is thought to be the best way of cooking kale. One cup of chopped kale has 30-40 calories and 684% of daily recommended intake of vitamin K, 206% of vitamin A and 134% of vitamin C.

High in:
Vitamin A
Vitamin C
Vitamin K
Manganese
Calcium
Copper

Kiwifruit:

Kiwi has more vitamin C than an equivalent amount of orange. It is believed that the anti-oxidants in kiwi can protect the DNA in cells. It may also be able to lower cholesterol and reduce the risk of heart disease. Kiwi may also reduce the risk of blood clots and reduce the fats in the blood. One medium kiwi has 40-50 calories and 117% of daily recommended intake of vitamin C.

High in:
Vitamin C

Vitamin K
Potassium
Fiber

Kohlrabi:

Kohlrabi is high in vitamin C and fiber but has no fat. It is in the cabbage family with a more delicate flavor. The entire plant is edible raw or cooked. The younger plants have an edible skin while the older tougher plants may need to be peeled. One cup of kohlrabi has 30-40 calories and 140% daily recommended intake of Vitamin C.

High in:
Vitamin C
Fiber
Vitamin B6
Potassium

Krachai:

Often referred to as fingerroot because of its shape the krachai is often found pickled in jars. It is believed that krachai can ease stomach troubles such as gastritis. It is also believed to boost energy and help cure eczema and ringworm. Krachai is believed to increase male libido.

High in:
Fiber

Kumquat:

Kumquats are eaten with the peel which adds fiber and essential oils. They are rich in vitamins and anti-oxidants. It is believed that kumquats may reduce the risk of certain cancers and degenerative diseases. They also contain minerals such as calcium and iron. One kumquat has 10-15 calories.

High in:
Vitamin C
Fiber

L

Lanzones:
Lanzones have some vitamins and minerals and no fat. It is believed that Lanzones can relieves diarrhea and reduce body temperature. A seven piece serving of Lanzones has 40 calories.

High in:
Vitamin C
Vitamin E

Leek:

Leeks are low in calories but high in vitamins and minerals. They also have anti-oxidants and fibers. Leeks may be able to lower blood pressure and prevent platelets from clotting. One leek has 30-40 calories.

High in:
Vitamin A
Vitamin K
Fiber
Iron
Sodium
Manganese

Lemon:

Lemons are high in vitamins but low in fat cholesterol and calories. Lemons have fiber and anti-oxidants. One lemon has 10-15 calories.

High in:

Vitamin C
Fiber

Lemongrass:

Lemongrass has essential, chemicals, minerals and vitamins that are thought to have anti-oxidant and disease preventing properties. It also has anti-microbial and anti-fungal properties. One cup of lemongrass has 60-70 calories and 175% of daily recommend intake of manganese.

High in:
Folate
Iron
Magnesium
Potassium
Zinc
Manganese

Lentils:

Lentils are one of the most nutritious and economical foods in the world. They are high in vitamins and minerals as well as fiber and protein. It is believed that lentils can reduce cholesterol and body weight. They are also believed to benefit digestion. Lentils are also thought to reduce the risk of breast cancer. One cup of cooked lentils has 220-240 calories.

High in:
Thiamin
Folate
Iron
Potassium
Copper
Manganese
Fiber

Protein

Lettuce:

Lettuce has very few calories but have vitamins, minerals and anti-oxidants. Lettuce is thought to protect the skin and eyes from ultra violet rays. It is believed that lettuce can help prevent age-related macular disease in the eyes. Lettuce in the diet is believed to prevent osteoporosis, iron-deficiency, cardiovascular and some cancers. The greener lettuces are more nutritious than the wither ones. One cup of shredded lettuce has 5-15 calories.

High in:
Vitamin A
Vitamin K
Vitamin C
Folate
Iron

Lime:

Limes are high in vitamin C and contain smaller amounts of other vitamins and minerals. Limes are thought to be anti-cancer and anti-bacterial properties. It is believed that taking lime juice once a day may help protect people from contracting cholera and kidney stones. One lime has 15-25 calories.

High in:
Vitamin C
Fiber

Longan:

It is believed that longans can treat stomach aches, infections and boost immunity. They are also believed to be calming to the nerves and an anti-depressant. Longans are believed to be beneficial to the blood in many ways. Traditionally longans are believed to reduce the effects of poison and have been used to treat snakebites. One longan has 1-3 calories.

High in:
Vitamin C
Magnesium
Phosphorus
Potassium

Lychee (Litchi):

Lychee has fiber, minerals, vitamins and anti-oxidants but no saturated fats or cholesterol. It is thought that lychee may help improve blood flow in organs, reduce weight and protect skin from UV rays. Lychee is believed to have anti-oxidant and anti-influenza properties. The seed is not poisonous but should not be eaten. One cup of lychee pulp has 120-130 calories and 226% daily recommended intake of Vitamin C.

High in:
Vitamin C
Vitamin B6
Copper
Fiber

M

Macadamia Nut:

Macadamia nuts are high in mono-unsaturated fats and contain vitamins, minerals and protein. They also contain anti-oxidants and may help with weight loss. Macadamia nuts are gluten free and are used in gluten free foods. Ten to twelve macadamia nuts have 200-205 calories.

High in:
Fat
Thiamin
Copper
Manganese
Fiber

Mace:

Mace enhances color, taste and flavor of foods and comes from the nutmeg tree. It has essential oils, vitamins and minerals. It is believed that mace has anti-fungal, anti-depressant, aphrodisiac and anti-cancer properties. It is also believed that mace helps with digestion. Traditional medicinal uses for mace include treating nervous system and digestive system illnesses. It has also been used to relieve pain in teeth and muscles. Mace has been mixed with honey to treat nausea, gastritis and indigestion. One tablespoon of mace has 20-30 calories.

High in:
Copper
Manganese
Vitamin C
Fiber

Fat

Malanga:

Malanga is a starchy vegetable similar to the potato but with hairy skin. It is not a significant source of vitamins, minerals, proteins or fats. Malanga should be cooked before eating. A one third cup serving of malanga has 60-80 calories.

High in:
Thiamine
Vitamin B6
Potassium
Phosphorus
Magnesium

Mango:

Mango is rich in pre-biotic fiber, vitamins, minerals and anti-oxidants. It is believed that mangoes can protect against colon, breast, leukemia and prostate cancers. Mango is also rich in alpha and beta carotenes. They also have potassium, B vitamins and copper. One cup of raw mangoes has 100-110 calories.

High in:
Vitamin C
Vitamin A
Vitamin B6
Potassium
Fiber

Mangosteen:

Because of the threat of the Asian fruit fly, mangosteen is often found canned in syrup. Mangosteen has been used to treat skin infections, dysentery and urinary tract infections. It is thought that mangosteen may reduce the risk of certain cancers. In traditional medicine, the mangosteen is believed to be good for the heart, help to keep youth, and have special effects for men and women. One cup of drained mangosteen has 140-145 calories.

High in:
Folate
Fiber
Manganese
Vitamin C

Maygrass:

Maygrass is native to the southeastern United States and Mexico. It is thought that maygrass made up part of the native diet as far back as 4000 years ago. Maygrass seeds are thought to be quite nutritious with a good amount of minerals and vitamins. Unfortunately there has been very little study of maygrass and thus little information.

Milk (cow):

Milk is high in vitamins, minerals and proteins. Fat free milk is fat free and low in cholesterol. Some verities of milk have vitamins A and D added. Milk is believed to be able to reduce the risk of atherosclerosis, certain cancers and hypertension. It is also believed that milk can improved immune system function and promote muscle growth and recovery. The trans-palmitoleic acid in dairy fat, found in milk, may reduce the risk of type 2 diabetes. Lactose intolerance in humans can cause diarrhea, intestinal gas, cramps and bloating. One cup of nonfat milk has 80-90 calories.

High in:
Calcium
Phosphorus
Riboflavin
Potassium
Protein
Vitamin B12

Millet:

Millet is low in calories and rich in vitamins and minerals. Millet is believed to be able to reduce cholesterol, high blood pressure and the risk of heart attack. It also believed that millet can reduce the risk of type 2 diabetes. They may also reduce the risk of gallstones and breast cancer in women. Millet may also protect against asthma in children. One cup of cooked millet has 205-215 calories.

High in:
Manganese
Copper
Phosphorus
Magnesium

Thiamin
Niacin
Protein

Mint:

Mint contains many vitamins and minerals. It has been used to aid digestion and as a healing compound. Used in cooking mint adds flavor without adding sodium. It is believed that min has anti-oxidant and anti-cancer properties. In traditional medicine mint is believed to clean the blood, clear acne, treat burns and itching, help breathing, relieve minor aches and relieves the symptoms of colds and flues. Two tablespoons of mint has 1-3 calories.

High in:
Vitamin A
Vitamin C

Mulberry:

Mulberries are low in calories and high in vitamins and minerals. It is believed that mulberries can reduce the risk of cancer, neurological diseases, inflammation, and infections. Mulberries are also thought to be good for eye health. One cup of mulberries has 55-65 calories.

High in:
Vitamin C
Vitamin K
Iron
Fiber

Mushrooms:

Mushrooms are low in calories, fat free, cholesterol free and gluten free. They are a good source of B vitamins and important minerals. Mushrooms are believed to be beneficial for the blood. They are also believed to boost the immune system and reduce the risk of cancer. Mushrooms also contain vitamin D, naturally. Some mushroom varieties are believed to have other effects on the body. One cup of white mushroom pieces has 10-20 calories.

High in:
Riboflavin
Niacin
Pantothenic acid
Copper
Potassium

Mustard Seed:

Mustard seeds are rich in essential vitamins which assist in lowering blood pressure. The anti-inflammation properties may also reduce the risk of gastrointestinal and colorectal cancers. Mustard seeds also have antifungal and antiseptic properties. Mustard is considered to have cleansing properties especially of the digestive system. Mustard seeds have also been used for clearing the lungs and boosting the body's metabolic rate. It is believed that mustard seeds can help treat mental disorders, such as depression and anxiety. One tablespoon of mustard seeds has around 32-45 calories.

High in:
Selenium
Curcumin
Magnesium

N

Nance:

Nance is high in fiber and low in calories. They can be eaten raw or cooked. One cup of nance has 80-90 calories.

High in:
Vitamin K
Vitamin   C
Manganese
Fiber

Nectarines:

Nectarines have low, but healthy, concentrations of important anti-oxidants. They are low in calories and have some vitamins and minerals. One cup of nectarine slices has 60-65 calories.

High in:
Vitamin C
Fiber
Potassium

Nungu:

Nungu or palm fruit is believed to have originated in India. Nungu provide a clean source of water and provide a good balance of minerals and sugar. Historically the Nungu has been used as a rejuvinative and tonic. It may also help with digestion. One hundred grams of Nungu has 35-45 calories.

High in:
Iron
Calcium
Vitamin B

O

Oats:

Oats are high in vitamins, minerals, fiber and protein. The fiber in oats is believed to be able to significantly reduce cholesterol levels. Oats are also believed to have unique anti-oxidants that can the risks of cardiovascular diseases. It is believed that oats can enhance the immune system and stabilize blood sugar. Oats are believed to reduce the risk of type 2 diabetes and some cancers. It is reported that oats can reduce the risk of childhood asthma. Some believe that whole grains, such as oats, have more health promoting activity than fruits and vegetables. One half cup of oats has 300-305 calories and 191% daily recommended intake of manganese.

High in:
Manganese
Phosphorus
Magnesium
Iron
Thiamin
Fiber
Protein
Folate
Copper
Zinc
Pantothenic acid

Okra:

Okra is low in calories and contains no saturated fats or cholesterol. Okra is rich in fiber, vitamins and minerals. Okra is thought to be able to relieve constipation and reduce the risk of some cancers. Okra is believed to have anti-oxidant properties. One half cup of okra has 15-25 calories.

High in:
Vitamin K
Vitamin C
Manganese

Olive:

Olives have anti-oxidant and anti-inflammatory properties. The hydroxytyrosol in olives are believed to prevent cancer and osteoporosis. Olives are high in monounsaturated fat which may reduce the risk of cardiovascular disease. Olives may also reduce blood pressure. One olive has 3-4 calories.

High in:
Iron
Fiber
Copper

Onion:

Onions are low in calories and fats but high in fiber. Onions are believed to have anti-mutagenic and anti-diabetic properties. They also release nitric oxide that reduces blood pressure. Onions are also believed to have anti-bacterial, anti-viral, and anti-fungal properties. Shallots are a type of onion that has small, elongated bulbs and a sweeter taste. One medium onion has 40-50 calories.

High in:
Vitamin C
Vitamin B6
Manganese
Fiber

Orange:

Oranges have no cholesterol or saturated fats and are low in calories. The fiber in oranges is thought to be able to reduce the cholesterol in the body. Oranges are believed to be able to reduce toxicity in the body and reduce the risk of some cancers. They are also believed to have anti-oxidant and anti-inflammatory properties. Oranges also contain alpha and beta carotenes. One cup of orange sections has 80-90 calories and 160% daily recommended intake of vitamin C.

High in:
Vitamin C
Fiber
Folate
Thiamin

P

Papaya:

Christopher Columbus reputably called the papaya the "fruit of the angels." The fruit is high in vitamins and minerals. The seeds are edible and have a peppery biter flavor. Papaya has been used to aid in digestion. They are believed to protect against heart disease and promote digestive health. Papaya is thought to have anti-inflammatory and anti-cancer properties. They are thought to boost the immune system and protect against macular degeneration disease. One medium papaya has 110-120 calories and 313% daily recommended intake of vitamin C.

High in:
Vitamin C
Vitamin A
Folate
Fiber
Potassium

Parsley:

Parsley is very high in vitamins and low in calories. Parsley is believed to have anti-inflammatory and anti-oxidant properties. Parsley is thought to be good for the heart and general health. It is also believed that parsley can reduce the risk of diseases such as rheumatoid arthritis. One half cup of parsley has 5-10 calories and 615% daily recommended intake of vitamin K.

High in:
Vitamin K

Vitamin C
Vitamin A
Folate
Iron

Parsnip:

Parsnips have vitamins, minerals and fiber. They also have the same anti-oxidants as carrots but with more sugar. Parsnips are a good source of dietary fiber. They are believed to have anti-inflammatory, anti-fungal, and anti-cancer properties. One half cup of parsnip slices has 50-60 calories.

High in:
Vitamin C
Fiber
Folate
Manganese

Pawpaw:

Pawpaw has vitamins, minerals, protein and fats. They have anti-oxidant and anti-fungal properties. The seeds and skin can be toxic in large quantities. One pawpaw has 70-90 calories.

High in:
Vitamin C
Riboflavin
Niacin
Potassium
Calcium

Peach:

Peaches have many vitamins and minerals but are low in calories and have no saturated fats. They have anti-oxidant properties and are believed to be good for the skin and eyes. Peaches have fluoride which is a component of bones and teeth and is believed to prevent tooth diseases. One large peach has 65-75 calories.

High in:
Vitamin C
Vitamin A
Potassium
Fiber

Peanut:

Peanuts are rich in energy, vitamins and minerals. They also contain protein, fiber and fats. Peanuts are believed to have anti-oxidant, anti-fungal, anti-viral and anti-cancer properties. They are also believed to reduce the risk of heart diseases, degenerative nerve disease, and Alzheimer's diseases. It is thought that boiling peanuts may increase the anti-oxidant properties. One half cup of dry roasted peanuts has 420-430 calories.

High in:
Manganese
Niacin
Magnesium
Phosphorus
Folate
Saturated Fat
Vitamin E
Potassium
Copper

Protein
Fiber

Pear:

Pears are high in anti-oxidants and low in calories. It is believed that the skin of the pear has more nutrition than the flesh. They are believed to improve insulin sensitivity. Pears may reduce the risk of type 2 diabetes, heart disease and some cancers. They also have anti-oxidant and anti-inflammatory properties. One small pear has 80-90 calories.

High in:
Vitamin C
Fiber
Vitamin K
Copper

Peas:

Peas have many vitamins and minerals, but contain no fat or cholesterol. They have anti-oxidant, anti-inflammatory and anti-cancer properties. Peas are believed to help regulate blood sugar and promote heart health. They are also environmentally friendly by adding nutrients to the soil. One half cup of peas has 55-65 calories.

High in:
Vitamin K
Vitamin C
Manganese
Fiber

Pecan:

Pecans are rich in energy, vitamins, minerals and anti-oxidants. They are high in monounsaturated fats that are believed to lower cholesterol. Pecans contain a number of nutrients that are believed to be powerful anti-oxidants. They also have anti-cancer properties. One cup of chopped pecans has 750-760 calories and 245% of daily recommended intake of manganese.

High in:
Thiamin
Fiber
Vitamin B6
Iron
Magnesium
Phosphorus
Potassium
Zinc
Copper
Manganese

Persimmon:

Persimmons are rich in health promoting vitamins, minerals and anti-oxidants. They are believed to have anti-infective, anti-inflammatory and anti-hemorrhagic properties. Persimmons are also believed to reduce the risk of age-related macular disease in the elderly. One fruit has 115-125 calories.

High in:
Vitamin A
Manganese
Vitamin C
Fiber

Pimento:

Usually found stuffed inside an olive, pimento provides vitamins and minerals on its own. Pimento is believed to have anti-oxidant, anesthetic, and analgesic properties. It is also believed to increase blood flow and relax nerves and muscles. Pimento has been used to help digestion and reduce gas. One tablespoon of pimento has 2-4 calories.

High in:
Vitamin C
Vitamin A

Pineapple:

Pineapple is an excellent source of vitamin C as well as other vitamins and minerals. They are believed to have anti-oxidants and anti-inflammatory properties. Pineapples are believed to boost the immune system and help digestion. They also may reduce the risk of age-related macular disease. One cup of pineapple chunks has 75-85 calories and 131% daily recommended intake of vitamin C.

High in:
Vitamin C
Manganese
Thiamin
Vitamin B6
Copper
Fiber

Pine nuts:

Pine nuts are rich in mono-unsaturated fats. They are believed to reduce cholesterol. Pine nuts are also believed to help reduce body weight. They are also gluten free. Ten pine nuts have 10-12 calories.

High in:
Manganese
Fat

Pistachio:

Pistachios are rich in many vitamins and minerals. They also contain proteins and fats. Pistachios are believed to have anti-oxidant and anti-toxin properties. They are believed to lower blood cholesterol and protect the body from cancers and infections. One half cup of pistachio nuts has 345-355 calories.

High in:
Manganese
Copper
Thiamin
Protein
Fiber
Vitamin B6
Phosphorus
Saturated Fat
Magnesium
Iron

Pitaya fruit:

Pitaya fruit is also known as the Dragon fruit. They have no cholesterol but do contain healthy monounsaturated fats. Pitaya are rich in anti-oxidants. It is believed that pitaya fruit can lower blood sugar levels and blood pressure. They may also have anti-cancer properties. It is thought that pitaya fruit can prevent memory loss and is beneficial for the skin, bones, teeth and eyes. One small pitaya fruit has 55-65 calories.

High in:
Vitamin C
Riboflavin
Niacin
Iron
Phosphorus
Vitamin A
Calcium
Fiber

Plantains:

Plantains are low in calories and have no fat, sodium or cholesterol. They are also rich in vitamins and minerals. Plantains that have black skins are fully ripe and the green skinned are partially ripe. Plantains are usually cooked because of the amount of starch they contain. Plantains have more vitamin C, vitamin A and potassium than bananas. One cup of plantain has 230-240 calories.

High in:
Vitamin A
Vitamin C
Vitamin B6
Folate
Magnesium

Potassium
Fiber

Plum:

Plums are rich in vitamin C and unsaturated fats. They also contain strong anti-oxidants. Plums are believed to increase the absorption of iron. One plum has 30-40 calories.

High in:
Vitamin C
Vitamin A
Vitamin K

Pomegranate:

Known as one of the "super fruits", the pomegranate is rich in nutrients and health promoting chemicals. The nutrients are contained in the small seeds that reside inside the pomegranate. They are believed to reduce cholesterol and boost immune system. Pomegranates are also believed to improve circulation and protect the body from cancer. They are also high in anti-oxidants. Pomegranates are also believed to reduce the risk of heart disease. One pomegranate has 230-240 calories.

High in:
Vitamin K
Fiber
Vitamin C
Folate
Copper

Pomelo, Pummelo:

Pomelo is considered the king of the citrus fruit kingdom for its size and vitamin C content. One serving of Pomelo has more than the daily recommend amount of vitamin C. Pomelo can be found in Asian markets and some large supermarkets. Pomelo contains pectin which is believed to purify the blood and reduced the risk of arterial deposits. The fruit is reported to lower cholesterol levels and help to regulate blood sugar. The active ingredients are found in the inner skin of the fruit. Eating too much of this fruit can cause constipation and kidney stones. A one cup serving has 70-80 calories and 193% of daily recommended intake of vitamin C.

High in:
Vitamin C
Iron
Fiber
Protein

Potato:

The vitamin C and potassium are found in the flesh of the potato while the fiber is found in the skin; it is best to consume the entire potato. Potatoes are high in anti-oxidants. A potato has 21 percent of the daily requirement for vitamin B6. Vitamin B6 is believed to help in cell growth, brain and nervous system support, and cardiovascular protection. Potatoes are low in calories if backed and topped lightly. One large potato has 270-300 calories and 121% of daily recommended intake of vitamin C.

High in:
Vitamin C
Thiamin

Vitamin B6
Niacin
Folate
Iron
Phosphorus
Potassium
Magnesium
Copper
Manganese
Fiber

Pumpkin:

Pumpkin has few calories and no cholesterol or saturated fats. They do have vitamins, minerals, fiber and anti-oxidants. Pumpkin provides one of the highest amounts of the essential vitamin A. The nutrients in pumpkin are thought to reduce the effects of aging on the skin and eyes. The seeds are high in fiber and offer over 100% of daily recommended intake of iron in one serving. The seeds are also rich in fatty acids, protein, and minerals. One cup of pumpkin has 45-55 calories and 245% of daily recommended intake of vitamin A.

High in:
Vitamin A
Vitamin C
Vitamin E
Riboflavin
Potassium
Copper
Manganese

Purslane:

Purslane is known in some parts of the world as a weed that troubles vegetable crops. However, purslane is rich in fatty acids, vitamins and other nutrients. It is also believed to help counter depression. Purslane has the highest amounts of omega 3 fatty acids than any other leafy vegetable. One cup of purslane has 5-10 calories.

High in:
Vitamin A
Vitamin C
Iron
Calcium
Magnesium
Manganese

Q

Quinoa:

Quinoa is a rich source of vitamins, minerals, proteins and unsaturated fats. The protein in quinoa is considered to be a complete protein. Quinoa also contains monounsaturated fat and omega 3 fatty acids. Quinoa is believed to have anti-inflammatory properties from multiple sources. Quinoa also has anti-oxidant and cholesterol reducing properties. Quinoa is gluten free and easily digestible. One half cup of quinoa has 110-120 calories.

High in:
Manganese
Magnesium
Phosphorus
Fiber
Copper

R

Radish:

Since ancient times, the Chinese have believed that eating radishes would immensely benefit overall health. They are low in calories and high in anti-oxidants, electrolytes, minerals, and fiber. It is believed that radishes have anti-cancer properties. Radishes are believed to help to detoxify the body. One medium radish has 1-2 calories.

High in:
Vitamin C
Folate
Potassium
Fiber

Rambutan:

Rambutan is low in fats and has a small amount of protein. They are thought to be good for the blood and help remove toxins from the body. Traditionally rambutan has been used to kill intestinal parasites, lesson the symptoms of diarrhea and treat fevers. One rambutan fruit has 5-10 calories.

High in:
Vitamin C
Niacin
Iron
Phosphorus

Rapini, broccoli rabe:

Rapini is low in calories but high in vitamin and minerals. It is believed that rapini has anti-oxidant, anti-inflammatory and anti-cancer properties. Rapini may also be beneficial to the eyes and may slow the progression of cataracts and macular degeneration disease. One cup chopped rapini has 8-10 calories and 112% daily recommended intake of vitamin K.

High in:
Vitamin K
Vitamin A

Raspberry:

Raspberries are high in vitamin and manganese, but also have lower amounts of many other vitamins and minerals. Raspberries have anti-oxidant and anti-inflammatory properties. They have the most effect when fully ripe. Raspberries are believed to have nutrients that can reduce obesity and blood sugar levels. They are also believed to reduce the risk of some cancers. One cup of raspberries has 60-70 calories.

High in:
Manganese
Vitamin C
Vitamin K
Fiber

Rhubarb:

Rhubarb has very few calories and no saturated fats or cholesterol. The stalks have many vitamins and minerals as well as anti-oxidants. It is believed that rhubarb can limit neuronal damage in the brain. One stalk of rhubarb has 5-15 calories.

High in:
Vitamin A
Vitamin K
Vitamin C
Manganese

Rice:

Rice is eaten as a staple and as filler around the world. Brown rice has many nutrients whereas the white rice has had many of the nutrients removed. Most white rice has been enriched with vitamins, but still does not have the same amount as the brown. One cup of brown rice has 680-690 calories and 346% of daily recommended intake of manganese.

High in:
Iron
Manganese
Magnesium
Selenium
Niacin
Vitamin B6

Rutabaga:

Rutabaga is low in calories and fat but rich in vitamins, minerals and fiber. They are thought to increase stamina and digestion. Rutabagas are also believed to reduce the risk of cataracts and support the capillaries. One cup of rutabaga cubes has 60-70 calories.

High in:
Vitamin C
Manganese
Potassium
Fiber
Phosphorus
Magnesium

Rye:

Rye is rich in many healthy nutrients such as vitamins, minerals. It also contains high levels of protein and fiber. Rye is believed to help with weight loss and reducing cholesterol levels. It may also reduce the risk of gallstones and type 2 diabetes. Rye is also thought to reduce cardiovascular disease and promote gastrointestinal health. It is believed to reduce the risk of some cancers, heart disease and childhood asthma. One cup of rye flour has 360-370 calories and 278% daily recommended intake of manganese.

High in:
Manganese
Fiber
Selenium
Phosphorus
Thiamin
Protein

S

Saffron:

Saffron gets its health benefits from plant derived chemical compounds instead of vitamins and minerals. It is believed to have anti-oxidant and disease preventing properties. Saffron has non-volatile compounds that reduce the risk of cancer, infections and immune diseases. In traditional medicines it has been used an antiseptic, antidepressant, anti-convulsant and to aid digestion. One tsp of saffron has 1-2 calories.

High in:
Manganese
Vitamin A

Sage:

In use since ancient roman times, sage is known for its health promoting and disease preventing properties. The essential oils in sage are believed to have counter-irritant, anti-inflammatory, anti-allergic, rubefacient, anti-fungal and anti-septic properties. Sage is also rich in vitamins and minerals. Sage is believed to enhance concentration and attention span. It is also thought to relieve grief and depression. One tablespoon of sage has 4-7 calories.

High in:
Vitamin K
Vitamin B6
Manganese
Calcium
Iron

Fiber

Sapodilla:

Sapodillas are rich in energy and help to revitalize the body quickly. The fiber in sapodilla is believed to relieve constipation and remove toxins from the colon. They are believed to have anti-oxidant, anti-inflammatory and anti-cancer properties. One sapodilla fruit has 140-150 calories.

High in:
Vitamin C
Fiber
Potassium

Seaweed:

Seaweeds provide many different vitamins and minerals as well as other benefits. The exact vitamins and minerals depend on the type, age and where the seaweed is grown. Seaweed is low in calories and fats. The main benefits of seaweed are cardiovascular and intestinal health. The fiber in seaweed is believed to bind with metals in the body such as mercury and lead and remove them from the body. One ounce of seaweed has 80-90 calories.

High in:
Manganese
Magnesium
Folate
Iron
Calcium
Zinc
Fiber
Thiamin

Riboflavin

Sesame:

Sesame seeds may be one of the oldest condiments. They are high in beneficial minerals and omega 6 essential acids. Sesame is believed to reduce cholesterol and blood pressure. It is also believed the sesame can be good for the bones, colon and brain. Sesame may also have anti-cancer properties. One tablespoon of sesame seeds has 90-100 calories.

High in:
Copper
Manganese
Iron
Calcium
Magnesium
Phosphorus

Sorghum:

Sorghum is gluten free and rich in fiber and protein. It has a high nutritional value and has anti-oxidant properties. Sorghum is also believed to reduce the risk of colon and skin cancers, lower cholesterol levels and promote cardiovascular health. One cup of sorghum has 650-651 calories.

High in:
Phosphorus
Carbohydrates
Fiber
Iron
Protein
Thiamin
Niacin
Potassium

Soybean:

Despite the controversy over soybean consumption, they do offer many important nutrients and health benefits. It is believed that the negative effects of soybeans may come from over processing. Soybeans are believed to reduce cholesterol levels and prevent some cancers. They are also thought to reduce the frequency of hot flashes in menopausal women. Soybeans are believed to promote bone health and may reduce appetite. They may also reduce the risk of type 2 diabetes and chronic obstructive pulmonary disease. One cup of soybeans has 290-300 calories.

High in:
Manganese
Protein
Vitamin K
Fiber
Iron
Phosphorus
Magnesium
Copper

Spelt:

Spelt is an ancient species of wheat, but has more protein. It has more vitamins and minerals then regular wheat and is more easily digested. Spelt may reduce the severity of arthritis, Lyme's disease, migraines, behavioral issues, skin irritations and irritable bowel syndrome if eaten regularly. One cup of spelt has 240-250 calories and 106% daily recommend intake of manganese.

High in:
Manganese

Fiber
Niacin
Phosphorus
Magnesium
Protein
Iron

Spinach:

Spinach has vitamins, minerals and powerful anti-oxidants. It also has anti-inflammatory and anti-cancer properties. It is believed that spinach can maintain bone density. One half cup of spinach has 3-5 calories.

High in:
Vitamin K
Vitamin A
Vitamin C
Manganese
Folate

Summer Squash:

Summer squash is very high in alpha-carotenes and anti-oxidants. The skin of the summer squash has a lot of the total anti-oxidants and fiber. Summer squash may have anti-inflammatory and blood sugar regulation properties. Historically dried summer squash seeds have been used for anti-microbial and anti-parasitic treatments and in support of the prostate. It is believed that eating summer squash may reduce the risk of some cancers. One cup of slice summer squash has 30-40 calories.

High in:
Fiber
Vitamin C

Magnesium
Potassium
Manganese

Star Anise:

Star anise is the star shaped fruit of an evergreen plant and is not related to true anise plants. It is one of the few sources of shikimic acid which has anti-viral properties. Star anise also has anti-fungal, anti-bacterial and anti-oxidant properties. One star anise has 20-25 calories.

High in:
Iron
Manganese
Copper
Magnesium
Calcium

Star fruit:

Star fruit is also known as carambola and is high in vitamins and fiber. It low in calories but high in anti-oxidants and is a good source of B-complex vitamins. Star fruit is believed to act as a diuretic, expectorant and to suppress cough. One cup of star fruit cubes has 35-45 calories.

High in:
Vitamin C
Fiber

Strawberry:

Strawberries are packed with vitamins, fiber and anti-oxidants. They have very high levels of anti-oxidants and more vitamin C than oranges. Strawberries are thought to protect the heart and lower cholesterol and blood pressure. They are also believed to guard against cancer. One large strawberry has 5-7 calories.

High in:
Vitamin C
Folate
Magnesium
Manganese
Potassium

Sunflower seed:

Sunflower seeds are rich in polyunsaturated fats, vitamins and minerals. They are believed to have anti-inflammatory and cholesterol lowering properties. Sunflower seeds are also believed to reduce the risk of cardiovascular diseases and can reduce the risk of cancer. They are believed to calm nerves, muscles and blood vessels. Sunflower seeds are believed to help detoxify the body. One ounce of sunflower seeds has 160-170 calories.

High in:
Vitamin E
Phosphorus
Manganese
Copper
Fat
Selenium
Fiber
Protein

Sweet Potato:

Sweet potatoes are one of the most nutritious and beneficial vegetables in the world. They are very high in vitamins and minerals. The sweet potato is very high in beta-carotene that may require a small amount of fat to digest properly. Sweet potatoes also have anti-oxidant and anti-inflammatory properties. They are also believed to help regulate blood sugar and reduce cholesterol levels. The skin of the sweet potato is edible and adds fiber. It is believed that steaming is the best way to prepare sweet potatoes. One cup of sweet potato has 170-190 calories and 769% daily recommended intake of vitamin A.

High in:
Vitamin A
Vitamin C
Manganese
Vitamin B6
Potassium
Fiber
Pantothenic acid
Copper
Niacin
Thiamin
Riboflavin

Swiss Chard:

Swiss chard originates from the Mediterranean area and was used by the Greeks and Romans for medicinal purposes. Though it comes in many different colors, the leaves and only the white colored stems are cooked and eaten. Swiss chard contains a unique blend of at least 13 different anti-oxidants. It is low in calories and is fat and cholesterol free. Swiss chard is one of the most nutritious vegetables on earth. Swiss chard is believed to have anti-oxidant, anti-inflammatory and blood sugar regulating properties. It is also believed to support bone health and detoxification of the body. One cup of Swiss chard has 6-8 calories and 374% daily recommended intake of vitamin K.

High in:
Vitamin K
Vitamin A
Vitamin C

T

Tapioca:

Tapioca is rich in carbohydrates and has no fat or cholesterol. It is believed to be able to increase circulation and red blood count. It is also thought that tapioca can improve digestion, lower cholesterol, improve the metabolism and maintain fluid balance. Tapioca is believed to prevent birth defects and Alzheimer's disease. One cup of dry tapioca pearls has 540-550 calories.

High in:
Iron

Taro:

Taro is fat, cholesterol and gluten free. Taro has vitamins, minerals and fiber. It is believed to reduce cholesterol levels and help skin and vision. One cup of cooked taro slices has 180-190 calories.

High in:
Manganese
Fiber
Vitamin B6
Vitamin E
Copper
Potassium

Tamarind:

Tamarind is rich in vitamins, minerals and fiber. The fiber in tamarinds is thought to detoxify and protect the colon. Tamarind also has anti-oxidant and anti-cancer properties. In traditional medicine has used tamarind as a laxative, digestive aid and remedy for intestinal problems. One cup of tamarind paste has 280-290 calories.

High in:
Thiamin
Magnesium
Potassium
Fiber
Iron

Tarragon:

Tarragon has one of the highest levels of anti-oxidants of any herb. It is believed to reduce the risk of heart attacks and strokes. Traditional medicine has used tarragon to stimulate the appetite, remedy for anorexia, flatulence and the hiccups. One teaspoon of tarragon has around one calorie.

High in:
Vitamin C
Calcium
Manganese
Iron

Tea:

Tea has many health benefits including anti-oxidants. It may also boost the immune system and brain activity. Tea is believed to fight cancer and heart disease, protect teeth and bones, and improve digestion. It may be able to reduce the risk of Alzheimer's disease. Tea is also believed to improve digestion, prevent food poisoning, and prevent dehydration. One cup of tea has 1-3 calories.

High in:
Manganese
Potassium

Teff:

Teff is the seed of an Ethiopian grass and is one of the smallest grains in the world. It is rich in vitamins, minerals and fiber. Teff is also high in amino acids and omega 3 fatty acids. Teff is a gluten free grain. The iron in teff is easily absorbed by the body. Teff is believed to be able to reduce blood sugar levels. One cup of teff has 708-720 calories and 892% of daily recommended intake of manganese.

High in:
Thiamin
Riboflavin
Niacin
Vitamin B6
Pantothenic Acid
Calcium
Iron
Magnesium
Phosphorus
Potassium
Zinc

Copper
Manganese
Selenium
Fiber

Tomatillo:

Tomatillos are low in calories but have vitamins, minerals and fiber. They have anti-bacterial and anti-cancer properties. Tomatillos may also be able to help control heart rate and blood pressure. They may also be good for the skin and eyes. One medium tomatillo has 10-12 calories.

High in:
Vitamin C
Vitamin K
Niacin
Magnesium
Fiber

Tomato:

Tomatoes are believed to be very good for heart. Studies have shown that tomatoes can lower cholesterol and prevent unwanted clumping of platelet cells in the blood. The Lycopene in tomatoes have been shown to promote the proper regulation of fats, especially in the bloodstream. The antioxidants in tomatoes may help have bone health and anti-cancer properties. Diets high in tomatoes have been linked with reduced neurological diseases and obesity. Some people may be allergic to tomatoes. One medium tomato has 22-30 calories.

High in:

Vitamin A
Vitamin C
Vitamin K
Lycopene
Potassium

Triticale:

Triticale is a hybrid of wheat and rye first bred in the 19th century. It was designed to combine the yield of wheat with the disease and environmental tolerance of rye. One cup of triticale has 640-650 calories and 308% of daily recommended intake of manganese.

High in:
Manganese
Protein
Thiamin
Folate
Pantothenic acid
Iron
Magnesium
Phosphorus
Zinc
Copper

Turmeric:

Turmeric is reported to reduce fat deposits, balance blood sugar and raise the metabolism. The key ingredient of turmeric is Curcumin which is said to cause fat cells to self destruct and reduces the formation of new fat cells. Curcumin has anti-oxidant and anti-inflammatory properties. Turmeric also strengthens the immune system and supports liver health. Turmeric is also believed to help joints and vision. It may also help reduce the risk of cancer. There is no reported toxicity to turmeric; however it may increase stomach acid. One tablespoon of turmeric has 20-30 calories.

High in:
Curcumin
Iron
Manganese

Turnip:

Turnips are high in protein and fiber, but low in sodium and sugar. The green leaves of the turnip are also high in nutrients such as beta carotene which is believed to reduce the risk for many diseases. It is believed that turnips maintain your liver so it metabolizes fat much better. Being low in calories and high in nutrition, turnips make a good food for weight loss. One medium turnip has 30-40 calories.

High in:
Vitamin C
Vitamin B6
Calcium
Potassium
Manganese
Fiber

V

Vanilla:

Ancient Mayans believed that vanilla had aphrodisiac properties. Vanilla may also contain anti-oxidant properties. One vanilla bean has 1-2 calories.

High in:
B complex vitamins
Calcium
Magnesium
Potassium
Manganese

W

Walnut:

It is believed that 90% of the phenols and other beneficial nutrients are in the skin of the walnut. Walnuts have an unusual and beneficial form of vitamin E. Walnuts are rich in anti-oxidants and anti-inflammatory properties. They are also very good for the heart and circulatory system. Walnuts are also high in omega 3 fatty acids. They may also reduce the problems in Metabolic Syndrome. Walnuts have anti-cancer properties and are though beneficial to those with diabetes type 2. One cup of chopped walnuts has 750-800 calories and 200% of daily recommended intake of manganese.

High in:
Thiamin
Vitamin B6
Folate
Iron
Calcium
Protein
Fiber
Magnesium
Phosphorus
Zinc
Copper
Manganese

Wasabi:

Wasabi has no fat or cholesterol. It is believed that wasabi has anti-cancer and detoxification properties. It is also believed to have anti-inflammatory and anti-bacterial properties. Wasabi is reported to relieve the symptoms of allergic reactions, asthma and arthritis. Wasabi is thought to reduce the risk of heart related diseases. One ounce of raw wasabi root has 25-35 calories.

High in:
Vitamin C
Magnesium
Potassium
Manganese

Wasabi Plant:

Wasabi is low in calories and has no saturated fats. Often called Japanese horseradish, the wasabi plant is actually a different species. Wasabi is difficult to grow and is often substituted outside of Japan. All of the wasabi plant is used. Wasabi is thought to have anti-bacterial and anti-oxidant properties. It is also used to remove toxins, stimulate the appetite and treat diarrhea. Wasabi is also used to clear clogged sinuses.

High in:
Vitamin C
Fiber

Water Chestnut:

Water chestnuts have no saturated fats, but do have omega-3 and omega-6 fatty acids. There are some vitamins and minerals in water chestnuts, but they are mostly just used for crunch in stir-fry's. One half cup of water chestnuts has 30-40 calories.

High in:
Vitamin B6
Potassium
Copper
Manganese

Watercress:

Watercress is high in nutrients but low in calories and fat. The seeds are also edible. It is very high in vitamin A and an excellent source of vitamin K. One cup of chopped watercress has 2-6 calories and 106% of daily recommended intake of vitamin K.

High in:
Vitamin A
Vitamin C
Vitamin K
Calcium
Copper

Watermelon:

Watermelons are rich in electrolyte and water. They are also high in anti-oxidants. Watermelons have more Lycopene than red tomatoes. One wedge of watermelon has 80-90 calories.

High in:
Vitamin C
Vitamin A
Potassium

Wheat (whole):

Wheat is a good source of fiber, protein, Vitamins and minerals. It is believed that a diet high in fiber and whole grains can help reduce a person's weight. Whole wheat may also reduce the risk of type 2 diabetes. Wheat is most often of the "red" variety; however there is now "white" wheat on the market which has a softer texture and a milder flavor. One cup of wheat flour has 400-410 calories and 228% of daily recommended intake of manganese and 121% of selenium.

High in:
Thiamin
Riboflavin
Niacin
Folate
Vitamin B6
Pantothenic Acid
Iron
Magnesium
Phosphorus
Potassium
Zinc
Copper
Manganese
Selenium

Wild Rice:

Wild rice is actually an aquatic grass and is more than likely to be cultivated instead of harvested wild. It has a good amount of vitamins and minerals and the protein is complete protein providing all the essential amino acids. Wild rice is gluten and sodium free. It contains 30% more anti-oxidants than white rice and has fewer calories. One cup of cooked wild rice has 150-170 calories.

High in:
Manganese
Zinc
Protein
Fiber

Winter Squash:

Winter squash is very high in alpha and beta carotenes. The seeds are edible and are high in omega 6 and omega 3 fatty acids if not over cooked. Squash plants absorb chemicals from the soil and can be used to remove contaminates, therefore it is best to by organically produced squash. Winter squash has a high level of anti-oxidants and anti-inflammatory properties. Winter squash may have benefits in cancer prevention and treatment. It is believed that winter squash may help regulate blood sugar levels. One cup of winter squash has 70-100 calories and 214% of daily recommended intake of vitamin A.

High in:
Vitamin A
Vitamin C
Vitamin E
Thiamin
Niacin
Vitamin B6

Folate
Magnesium
Potassium
Manganese

X

Ximenia:

Ximenia is a semi-deciduous tree found all over Africa. All parts of the tree are used, from the leaves and bark to the roots and fruit. The fruit is high in vitamin C and can be used fresh or in preserves. The bark is used to treat stomach aches, mouth infections and toothaches. The leaves are used to treat nightmares. One Ximenia fruit has 40-60 calories.

High in:
Vitamin C

Y

Yam:

There are around 200 varieties of yams and are not to be confused with sweet potatoes. It is believed that the nutrients in yams can reduce the risk of cardiovascular disease. Historically yams have been used for kidney health and to support women's bodies. One cup of cubed yams has 150-160 calories.

High in:
Vitamin C
Vitamin B6
Potassium
Copper
Manganese

Yautia (tannier):

Yautia is similar to potato and malanga. It is not a significant source of vitamins, minerals, proteins or fats. One cup of sliced yautia has 130-145 calories.

High in:
Potassium
Vitamin B6
Copper
Manganese
Vitamin C

Yogurt (plain, skin milk):

Yogurt is low in fat and high in nutrients. The calcium and vitamin d in yogurt may prevent against bone diseases such as osteoporosis. Yogurt also has beneficial bacteria that can help protect your digestive tract. The bacteria in yogurt may help with lactose intolerance, constipation, diarrhea, colon cancer, and inflammatory bowel disease. Yogurt may also help in lowering blood pressure. The active cultures in yogurt may reduce the risk of vaginal infections. Yogurt being made from milk is also high in protein. One cup of yogurt has 130-140 calories.

High in:
Riboflavin
Vitamin B12
Calcium
Magnesium
Phosphorus
Potassium
Zinc
Selenium

Yucca:

Yucca root, also known as cassava, is low in fat and high in vitamins and minerals. Yucca is low in fat and cholesterol free. Yucca may reduce the risk of heart disease, stomach cancer and high blood pressure. One cup of yucca has 310-340 calories.

High in:
Vitamin C
Niacin
Iron
Calcium

Manganese

Yuzu fruit:

Yuzu is a hybrid of mandarin and papeda cultivated in the Far East. It is rich in anti-oxidants and is believed to have a fat burning effect. Yuzu is used for culinary purposes and as a fragrance. It is thought to promote relaxation and recovery of muscles. Yuzu is also thought to be good for the skin. One yuzu fruit has 20-30 calories.

High in:
Vitamin C
Potassium

Anti-oxidants

Oxygen is required for the vast majority of life on the planet. However oxygen is a very reactive molecule that can damage living organisms. Using oxygen in day to day activities create free radicals through oxidation.

Oxidation is a chemical reaction that transfers electrons from a substance to an oxidizing agent. Oxidation can produce free radicals which can then start chain reactions. When chain reactions occur in cells it can damage or kill the cell, it may even alter the DNA in a cell. The chain reactions in cells cause oxidative stress which can damage cell structure and cell function. Oxidative stress can cause excessive inflammation and seems to play a significant role in many diseases including cancer.

Anti-oxidants terminate chain reactions of free radical by being oxidized themselves, thus stopping the reaction. Anti-oxidants are used by nearly all plants and animals to protect themselves from these chain reactions. The anti-oxidants found in foods and supplements may help prevent diseases such as cancer, coronary heart disease, stroke, Alzheimer's, rheumatoid arthritis and cataracts.

It is best to get anti-oxidants from food instead of supplements. Anti-oxidants are abundant in beans, grains and brightly colored fruits and vegetables. Lutein is a yellow/orange colored anti-oxidant found in corn, squashes, etc. Lycopene is a red colored anti-oxidant found in tomatoes and watermelons. Flavonids/polyphenols the purple/blue anti-oxidants in berries, grapes, tea and wine are also very important.

Nutrients

Vitamin A

Vitamin A is good for growth, the immune system, reproduction and vision. It is also known to play an important role in bone growth and cell division. Vitamin A is an anti-oxidant and helps protect against cancer and other diseases. It also helps the body retain moisture preventing dry skin. Vitamin A may help in getting rid of aging lines and spots, giving the skin a younger appearance. Vitamin A in the form of beta-carotene can be found in orange and dark green vegetables.

Found in:
Carrots
Kale
Mangos
Pumpkin
Sweet potatoes
Winter squashes

Vitamin B

A group of water soluble vitamins that were one thought to be a single vitamin, however it is now believed that there are eight different chemically distinct vitamins that coexist as B vitamins. Foods containing all eight vitamins are referred to be vitamin B complex.

B complex vitamins can be found in:
Whole grains

Thiamine (B1)

B1 plays a central role in getting energy from carbohydrates and producing RNA and DNA. B1 is important for the heart, muscles and the nervous system.

Riboflavin (B2)
B2 is involved with energy production for the electron transport chain, the citric acid cycle and the catabolism of fatty acids. B2 is important for growth and the development of red blood cells.

Niacin (B3)
B3 plays an important role in energy transfer in the metabolism of sugar, fat and alcohol. B3 is important for digestion, skin and nerves.

Pantothenic Acid (B5)
B5 is important for the oxidation of fatty acids and carbohydrates. B5 assists in growth and metabolism.

Pyridoxine (B6)
B6 is involved in the metabolism of amino acids and lipids. B6 is important for the proper functioning of the immune system, nervous system, cell growth and blood sugar regulation.

Biotin (B7)
B7 is important in the metabolism of lipids, proteins and carbohydrates. B7 also assists in growth.

Folic Acid / Folate (B9)
B9 is involved in the metabolism of nucleic acids and amino acids. Folate is needed for proper cell division and the production of red blood cells.

Cobalamin (B12)

B12 is involved in the metabolism of carbohydrates, proteins and lipids at the cellular level. It is essential in the production of bone marrow and nerve sheaths.

Vitamin C

Vitamin C is one of the safest and most effective nutrients. It may help protect against immune system and cardiovascular diseases as well as eye and skin problems. Studies have shown that the RDA recommendation for vitamin C is far too low; with vitamin C, more is better. Vitamin C may reduce the length of colds and their severity; it may even keep you from getting a cold. It may also prevent lead poisoning and cancer. Some studies have suggested that vitamin C may even be able to lower cholesterol and blood pressure. It is thought that exposure to oxygen can destroy vitamin C.

Found in:
Guava
Jicama
Kale
Kiwifruit
Lychee
Oranges
Papaya
Peppers
Pineapple
Pomelo
Potato

Vitamin D

Vitamin is needed for the proper absorption of calcium and phosphorus. Aids in bone and tooth function.

Found in:
Sun exposure

Vitamin E

Vitamin E is believed to support the heart and blood vessels. It may reduce the risk of heart attacks and hardening of the arteries. Vitamin E is also used for treating diabetes and its complications. Vitamin E may also be used for cancer prevention, including lung, oral, colorectal and gastric cancers. It is also an anti-oxidant which has numerous anti-aging benefits for the body. Vitamin E is believed to regulate Vitamin A in the body.

Found in:
Almonds
Asparagus

Vitamin K

Vitamin K plays a major role in blood clotting. It may also help maintain strong bones in the elderly. Vitamin K may also be able to treat cystic fibrosis, heart disease and high cholesterol. It is believed that vitamin K can affect the rate at which some medications are absorbed.

Found in:
Dandelion
Endive
Kale
Parsley
Rapini
Swiss chard
Watercress

Calcium

There is more calcium in your body than any other mineral. Calcium helps in building stronger and denser bones. It also keeps bones stronger later in life. Calcium is needed for proper contraction of muscles, especially the heart. It has been believed that high intake of calcium may contribute to kidney stones. There are studies that show high intake of calcium may reduce the risk of kidney stones.

Found in:
Beans
Broccoli
Figs
Kale
Nuts
Okra
Quinoa
Seaweed

Copper

Copper is needed for the production of red blood cells. It also helps the blood vessels, nerves and immune system.

Found in:
Beans
Leafy greens
Nuts
Potatoes
Whole grains

Fatty Acids

Fatty acids are usually derived from triglycerides or phospholipids. They are an important fuel because they yield large amounts of ATP when metabolized. ATP is important as an energy transportation coenzyme. Omega 3 and omega 6 are considered essential because the body cannot produce them. Fatty acids are used by the heart, skeletal muscles and brain. Fatty acids are believed to reduce inflammation and the risk of chronic diseases such as cancer and heart disease. The brain has large amounts of fatty acids that are used for cognitive and behavioral functions. It is important to have the correct balance of omega 3 and omega 6 fatty acids. It is believed that modern humans get far too much omega 6. The proper ratio is believed to be near 1 to 1.

Omega 3 Found in:
Brussels sprouts
Fish
Flaxseed
Garlic
Kale
Mint
Oatmeal
Peanuts
Spinach
Walnuts
Watercress
Whole grains

Omega 6 Found in:
Meat
Poultry
Safflower oil
Sunflower seeds

Walnuts

Fiber

Fiber is an indigestible carbohydrate. Fiber adds bulk to keep you feeling full longer. It can also help regulate blood sugar. Soluble fiber dissolves in water and helps lower blood glucose and blood cholesterol levels. Insoluble fiber does not dissolve in water and helps move food through the digestive system. Fiber may also reduce the risk of gallstones. The liver uses cholesterol to create bile for emulsifying the fats we eat. Some fibers bind together with bile in the intestines and pass it out of the body. This means that the liver needs to make more bile thus using more cholesterol.

Found in:
Beans
Jicama
Whole Fruits
Whole grains
Whole vegetables

Iron

Iron is required for red blood cell formation. Iron helps with the transmission of oxygen throughout the body. Iron is part of many enzymes used by the body.

Found in:
Beans
Leafy greens
Whole grains

Manganese

Manganese is an essential mineral that the body needs to process fats, carbohydrates and proteins properly. Manganese along with copper, zinc and copper may help strengthen bones. It is also involved in thyroid function, sex hormone function, blood sugar regulation and immune function. Manganese may also help reduce the symptoms of Premenstrual syndrome, anemia and arthritis.

Found in:
Amaranth
Buckwheat
Hearts of palm
Lemongrass
Oats
Pecan
Rice
Rye
Spelt
Teff
Triticale
Walnut
Wheat

Magnesium

Magnesium is important to nearly every function of the human body. It is important for the proper contracting and relaxing of muscles. Magnesium also helps in the production protein and the transport of energy. It is also important to enzymes in the body. Magnesium may also be able to raise cognition in Alzheimer's patients.

Found in:
Avocados
Beans
Nuts

Peas
Whole grains

Phosphorus

Phosphorus is important for the formation of bones and teeth. It plays an important role in the growth of cells and tissues. Phosphorus is also involved in the storage of energy in the form of ATP. Phosphorus works with B vitamins and assists in the contraction of muscles and the functioning of the kidneys. It is also important in regulating heart beat and in supporting nerve condition.

Found in:
Beans
Whole grains

Potassium

Potassium is used to break down and use carbohydrates and build muscle and proteins. It is also used to maintain normal body growth and the acid-base (PH) balance. Potassium is used to control the electrical activity of the heart. It may also help to maintain normal blood pressure.

Found in:
Apricots
Beans
Beets
Potatoes
Soybeans
Squash

Selenium

Selenium is a trace mineral that is used to create anti-oxidant enzymes that prevent cell damage. It also supports the immune system. Selenium may help in reducing the risk of certain cancers and cardiovascular disease. It may also protect the body from heavy metal poisoning.

Found in:
Garlic
Mushrooms
Onion
Wheat
Whole grains

Sodium

Sodium regulates water and electrolyte balance and is required for nerve and muscle activity. It also maintains a regular acid-base (PH) balance. Sodium helps with the absorption of water and some nutrients. It also controls blood pressure and blood volume. It is believed that too much sodium may cause high blood pressure.

Found in:
Celery
Processed foods
Salt
Seaweed

Sulfur

Sulfur is believed to be good for the hair, skin, nails and connective tissue. It may be used in metabolism and in joint health.

Found in:
Beans
Cabbage
Nuts
Onions

Zinc

Zinc is an important trace mineral used by the body's immune system. It is also plays a role in cell division, cell growth and the breakdown of carbohydrates. Zinc is also needed for smell and taste. Zinc may reduce the risk of becoming sick. Taking zinc when first feeling ill may reduce how long and how severe a cold may be.

Found in:
Beans
Seaweed
Whole grains

Phytonutrients

Phytonutrients are natural chemicals found in plants that are believed to be beneficial to humans. These chemicals protect the plants from bugs, fungi and other threats. Phytonutrients can be found in fruits and vegetables, grains, nuts and tea.

Phytonutrients are not essential as vitamins and minerals are. They are believed to be beneficial to humans and may prevent diseases and keep the body operating properly. There are more than 25,000 phytonutrients found in plants but not all are considered beneficial.

Carotenoids, Ellagic acid, Flavonids, and Glucosinolates are some of the important phytonutrients found in plant and are thought to have health benefits. Carotenoids provide yellow, orange and red colors and act as anti-oxidants. They are found in carrots, tomatoes and squash. Ellagic acid is found in berries and other foods and is believed to protect against cancer.

Flavonids are a large category of nutrients. Catechins are flavonids found in green tea that may prevent certain types of cancer. Hesperidin is found in citrus fruits and has anti-oxidant and anti-inflammatory properties. Quercetin is a well studied flavonol found in apples, berries, grapes and onions. It may reduce the risk of asthma, certain types of cancers and coronary heart disease.

Glucosinolates are found in cruciferous vegetables such as Brussels sprouts, cabbage, broccoli and kale. Glucosinolates change into other chemicals during cooking and digestion. These chemicals may stunt the development and growth of cancer.

Polyphenols

Polyphenols are a type of anti-oxidant created in response to ecological pressures. These pressures include pathogen or insect attack, UV radiation or physical damage. The polyphenols found in foods are naturally occurring.

Capsaicin, found in chilies, is believed to have cancer preventing and fighting properties. Carvacrol, found in oregano, is believed to have anti-microbial and neuroprotectant properties. Other polyphenols such as salicylic acid and cannabinoids are used to relieve pain. Some polyphenols add flavors to foods. Others are antiseptics such as thymol, found in thyme.

Polyphenols may have beneficial effect on the body. Evidence for the role of polyphenols in the prevention of diseases such as cancer and cardiovascular disease is continuing to emerge. They are not simply anti-oxidants and are still being actively researched.

It is believed that long term consumption of polyphenol rich foods may reduce the risk of diseases such as, cancer, diabetes, osteoporosis, cardiovascular and neurodegenerative disease. Fruits such as grapes, apple, pear and berries have large amounts of polyphenols. Any products of these fruits would also have polyphenols. Many other fruits and vegetables have polyphenols as do seasonings.

www.ingramcontent.com/pod-product-compliance
Lightning Source LLC
Chambersburg PA
CBHW070142290526
45789CB00002B/596